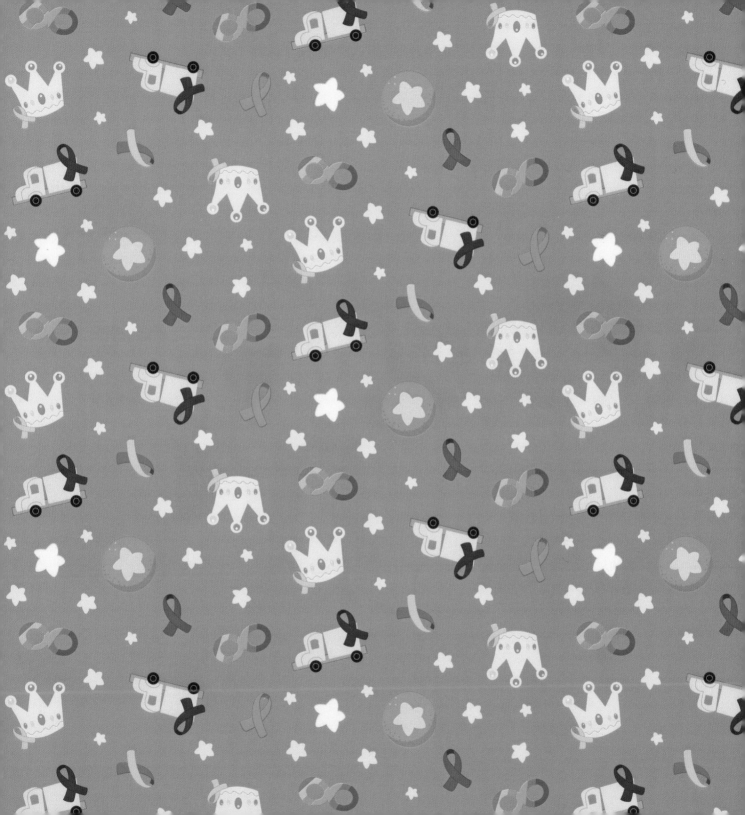

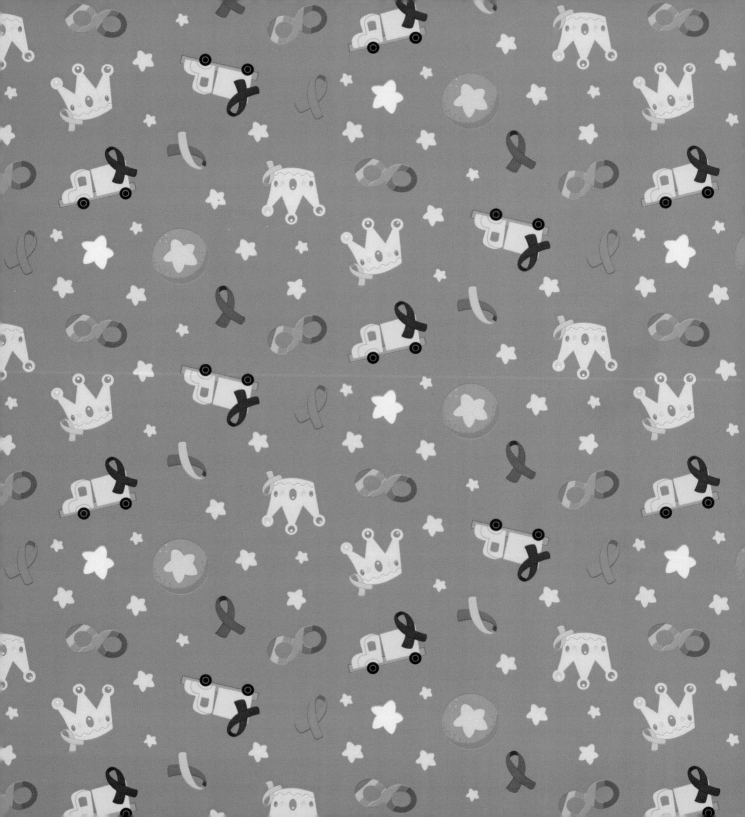

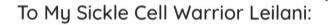

To My Sickle Cell Warrior Leilani:

I want you to know that you have inspired me more than you will ever know. Your strength to overcome at such a young age has made me a better person.
I am honored and blessed to be your mother.
I love you.

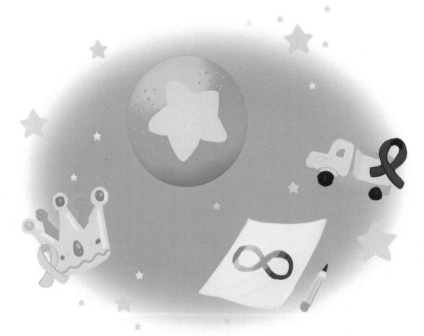

Braver Than I May Know by Grace Holloman

Book #1 in the *Braver Than I May Know* series

Copyright © 2022 Grace Holloman

A portion of the proceeds from Braver Than I May Know will be donated to The Jimmy Everest Center for Cancer and Blood Disorders at OU Children's Hospital in Oklahoma City, Oklahoma.

Illustrated by Shiane Salabie

Registration Number: TXu 2-280-919

ISBN: 978-1-66784-666-8

Printed in the United States of America.

BRAVER THAN
I MAY KNOW

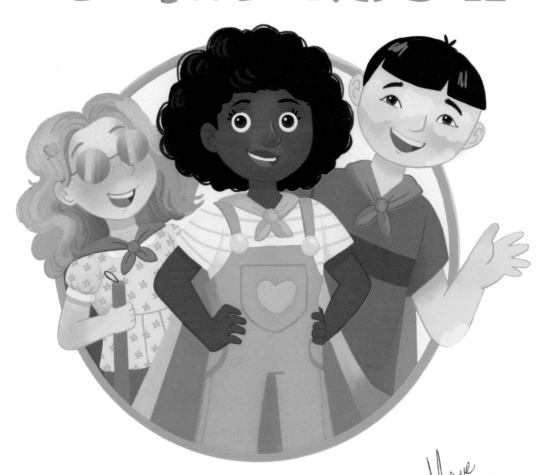

Written by **Grace Holloman**

Illustrated by **Shiane Salabie**

I am braver than I may know,

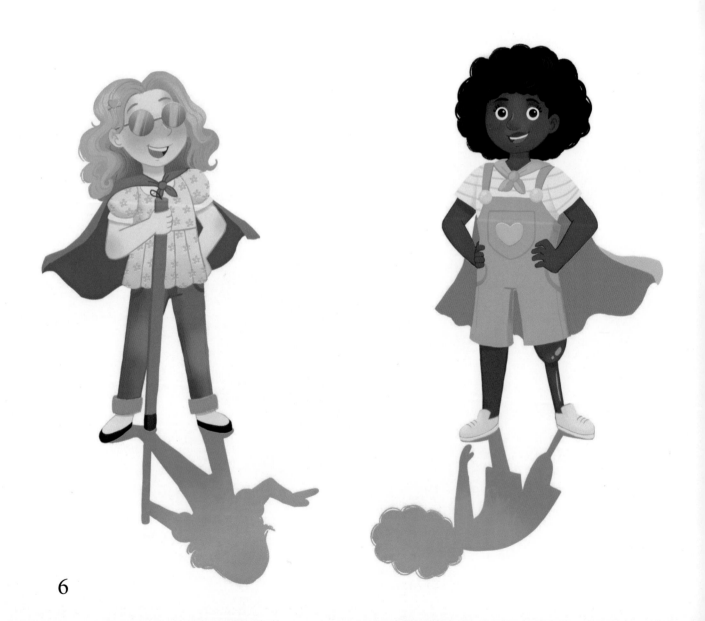

Stronger than I may feel . . .

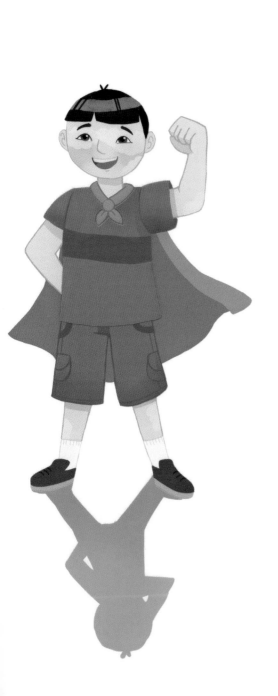
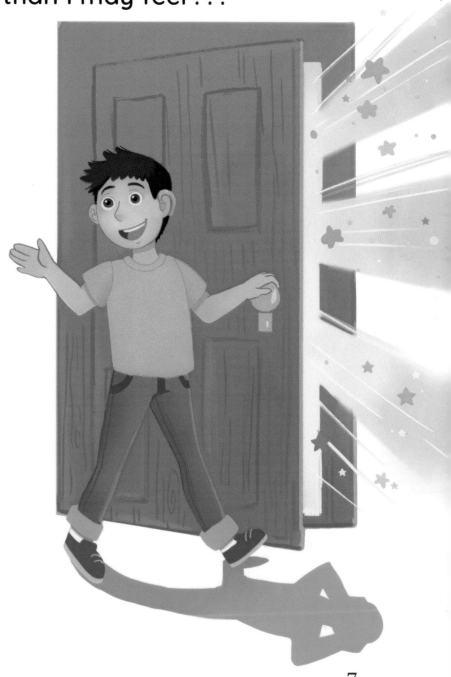

I may have a sickness that wears me down,

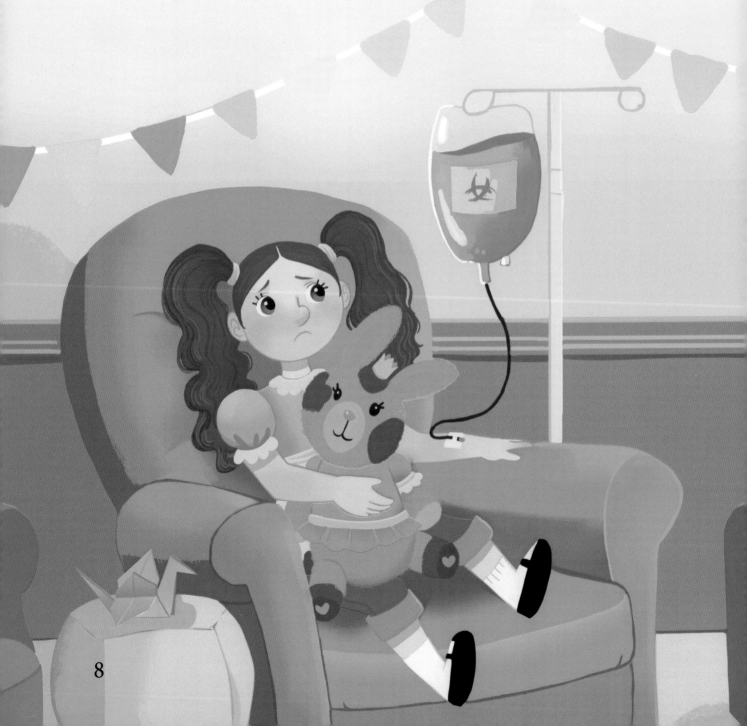

8

I may lose my hair, but I still wear a crown.

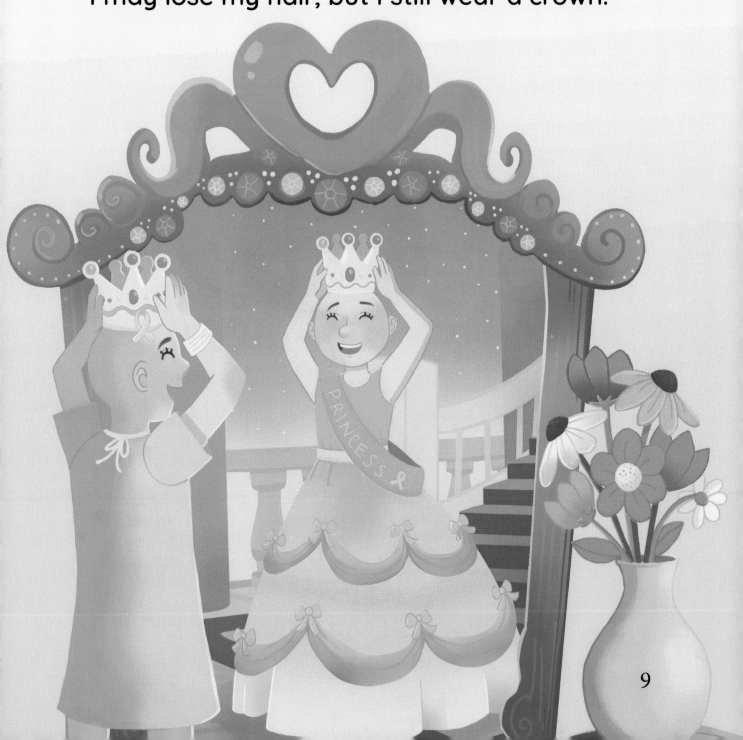

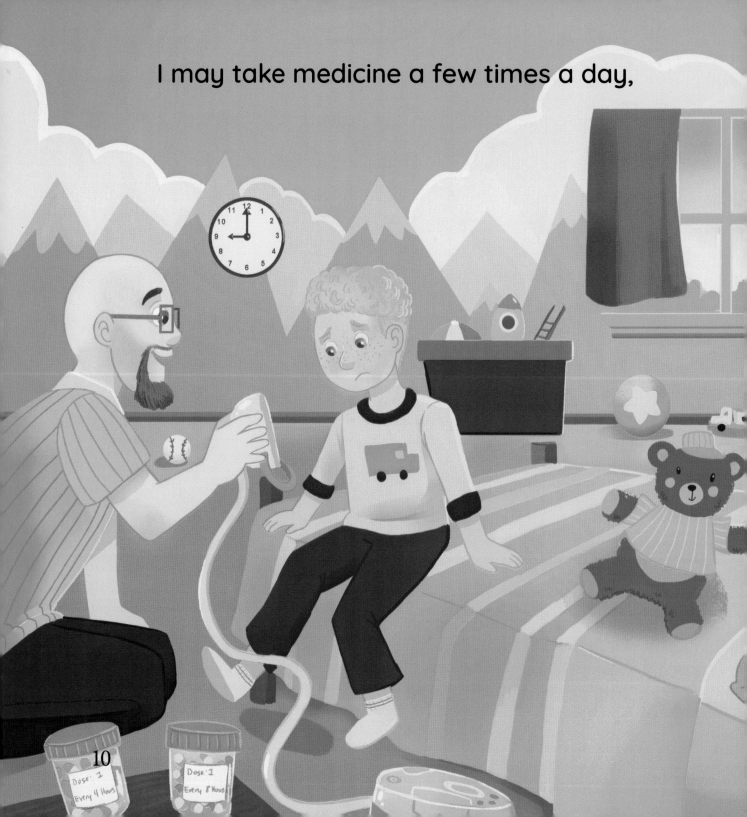

I may take medicine a few times a day,

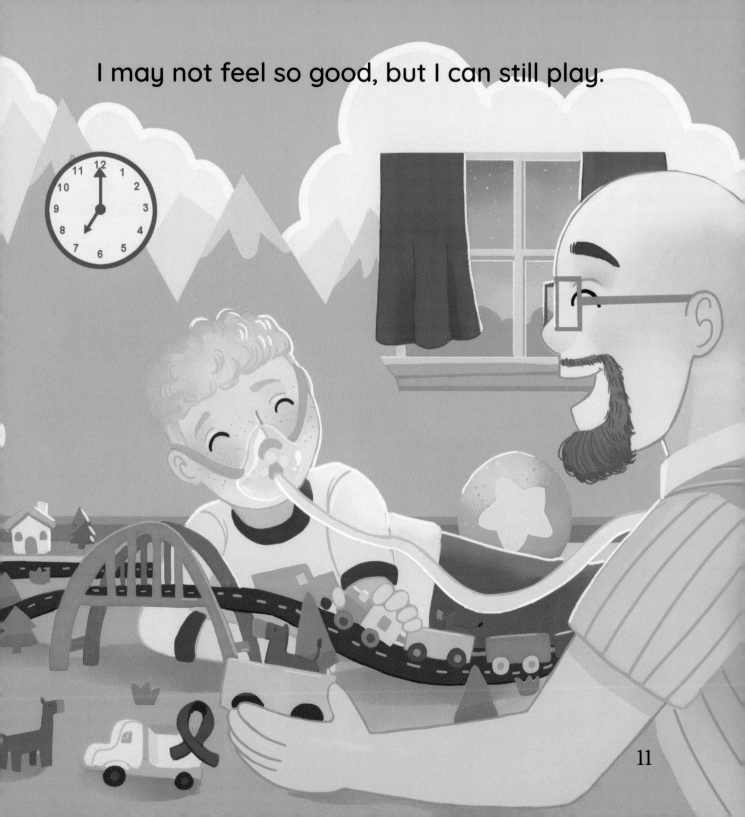

I may not feel so good, but I can still play.

11

I may have to miss a few days of school,

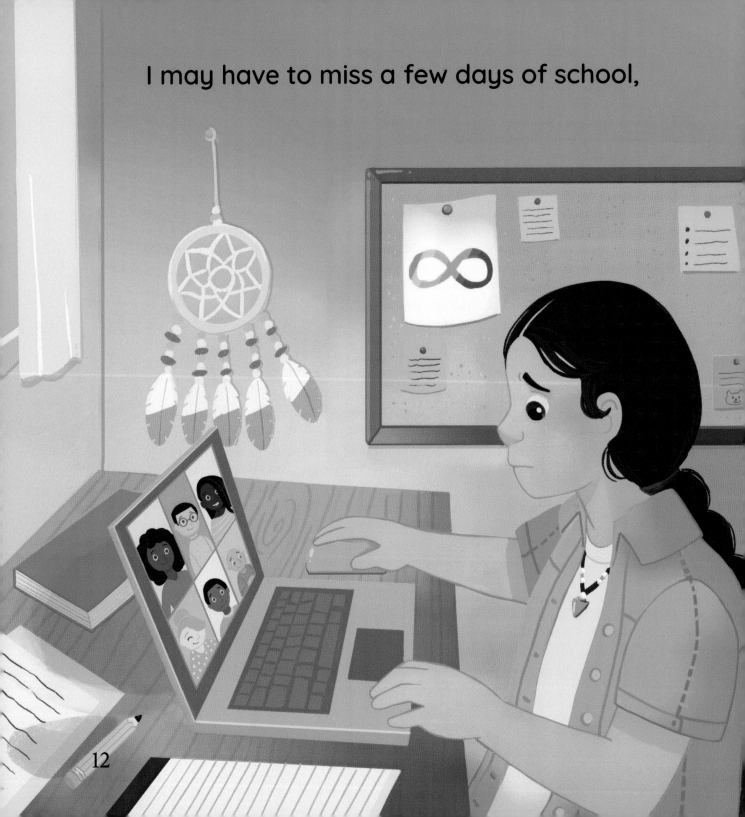

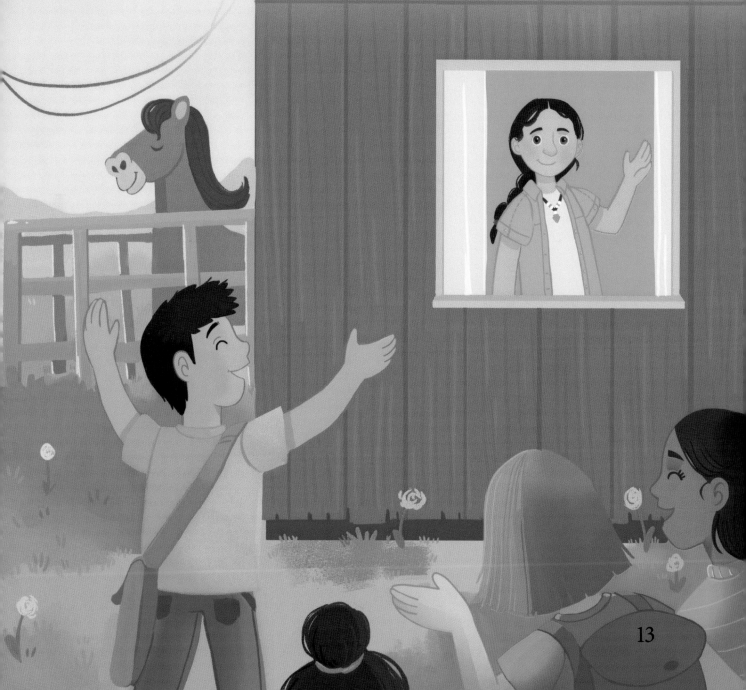

I may miss hanging out with my friends,
but they still think I'm cool.

13

I may be stuck inside for hours at a time,

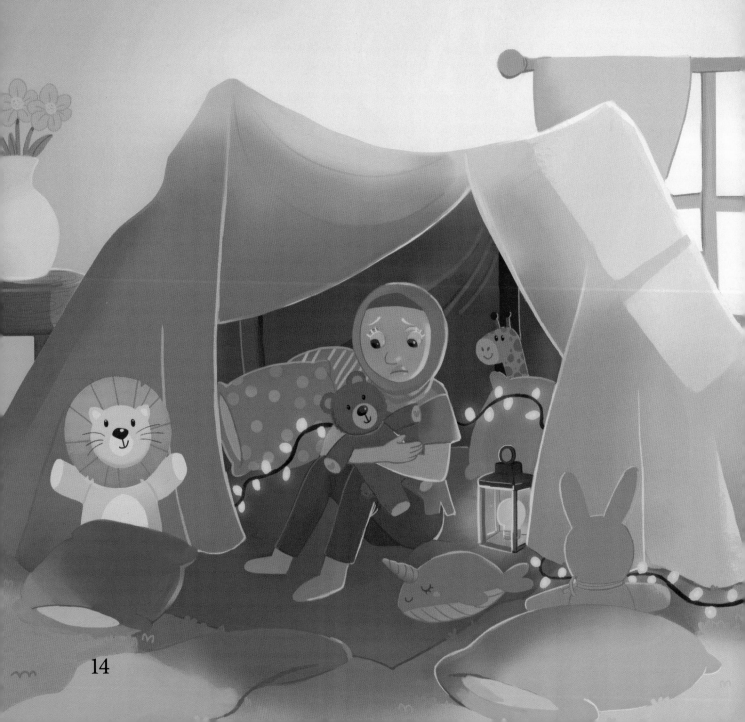

I may miss walking in the sun, but
I can still shine.

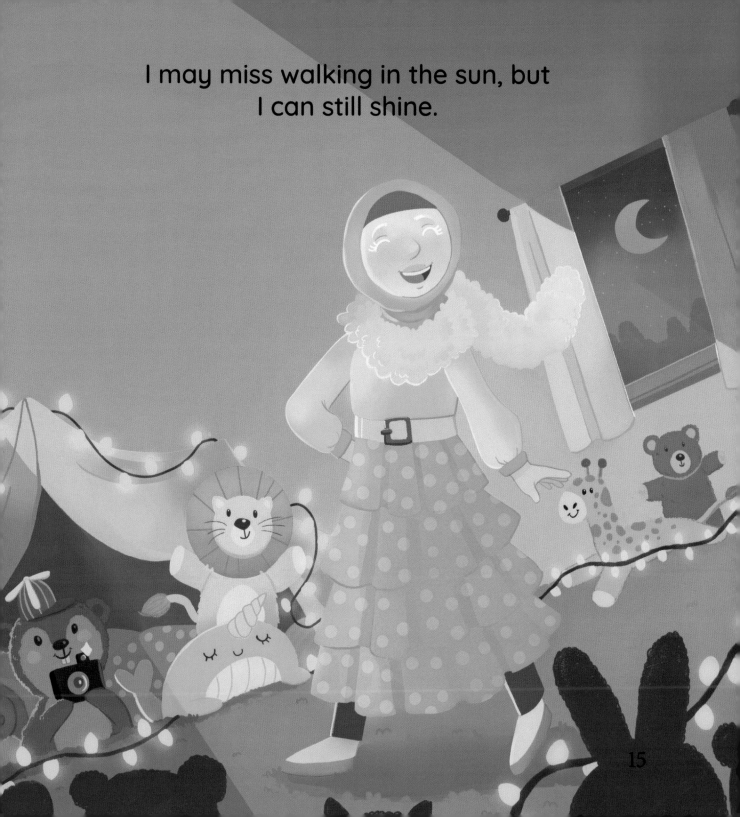

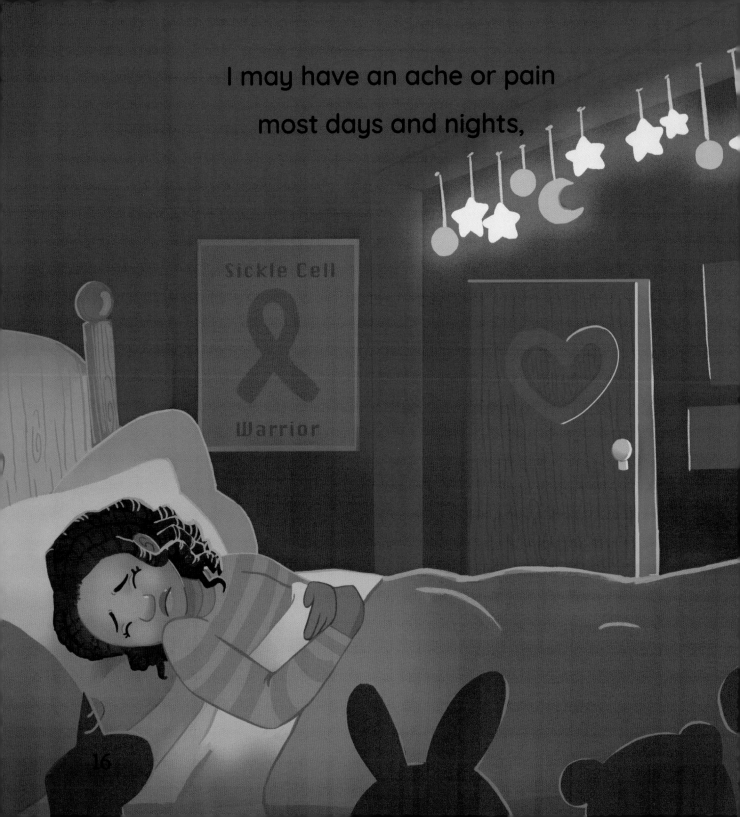

I may have an ache or pain
most days and nights,

I may be sad about it, but I feel better when mom and dad hold me tight.

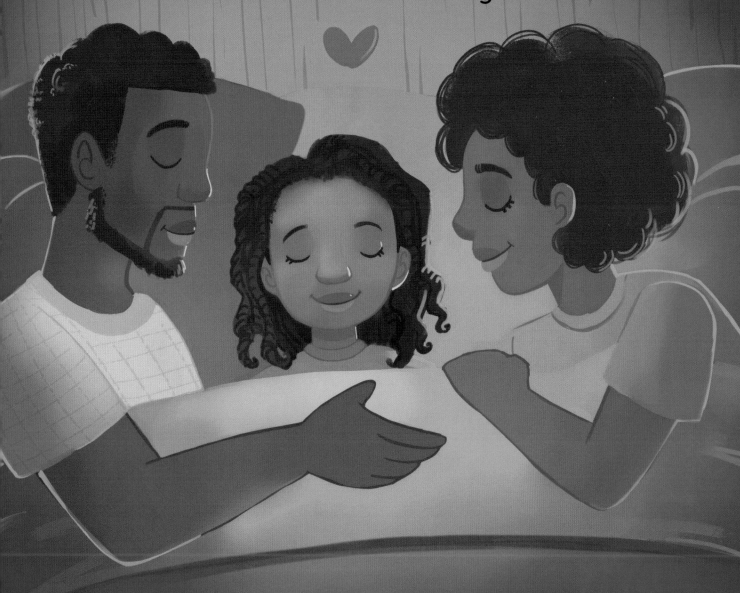

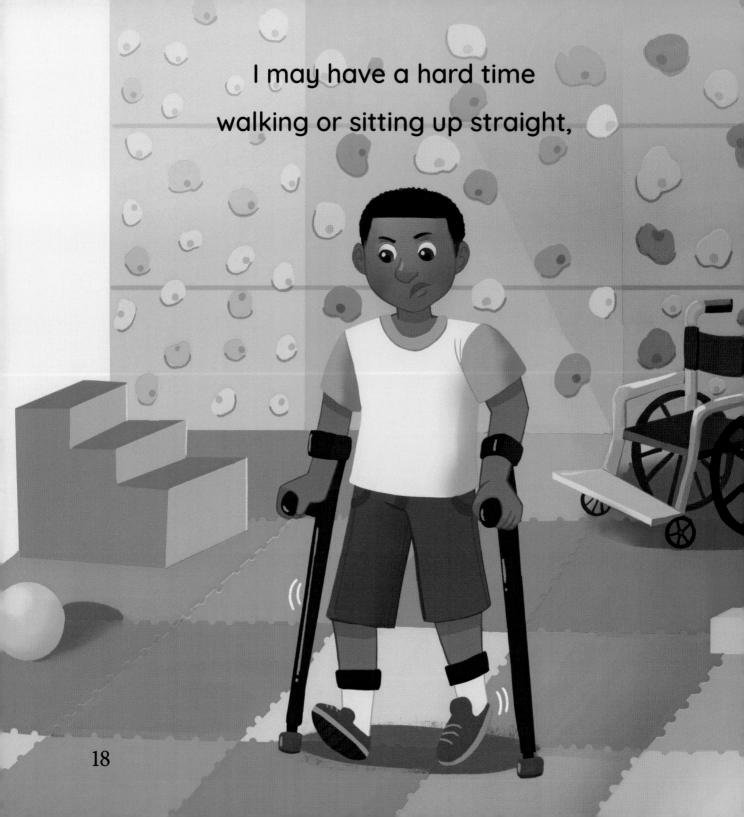

I may have a hard time
walking or sitting up straight,

18

I may fall down sometimes, but
I can still create.

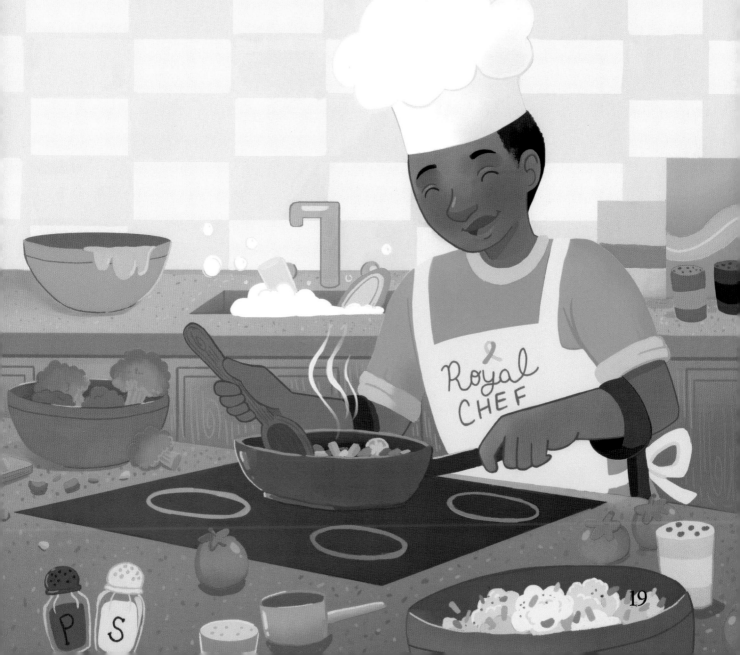

19

I may have doctor appointments, some I would not choose,

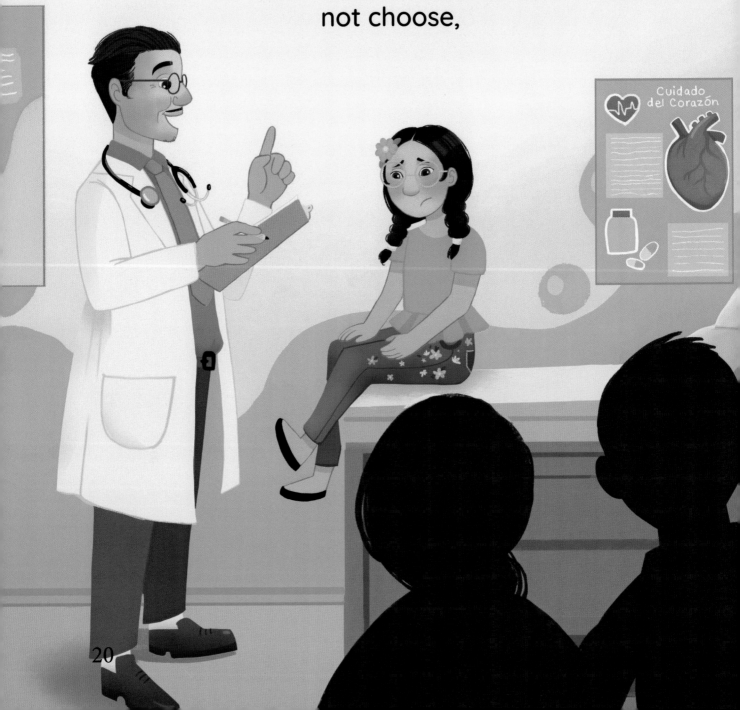

I may not always feel like fighting, but I refuse to lose.

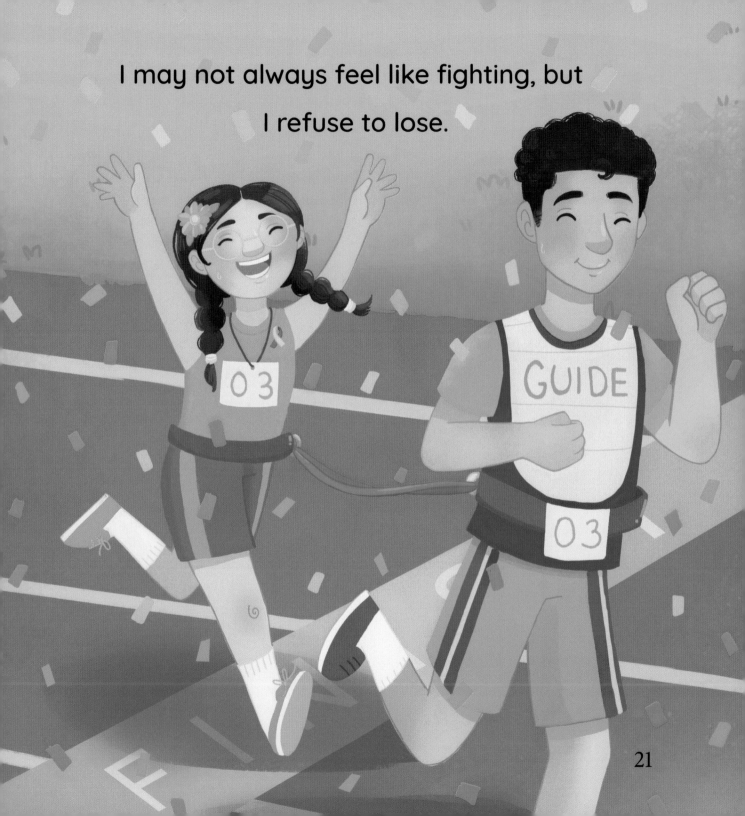

I am braver than I may know,

Stronger than I may feel,

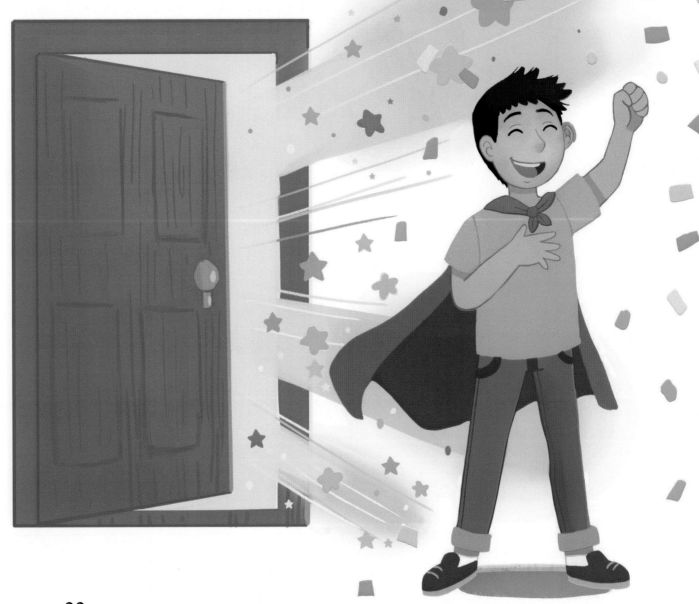

I am a warrior,

a fighting spirit lives within!

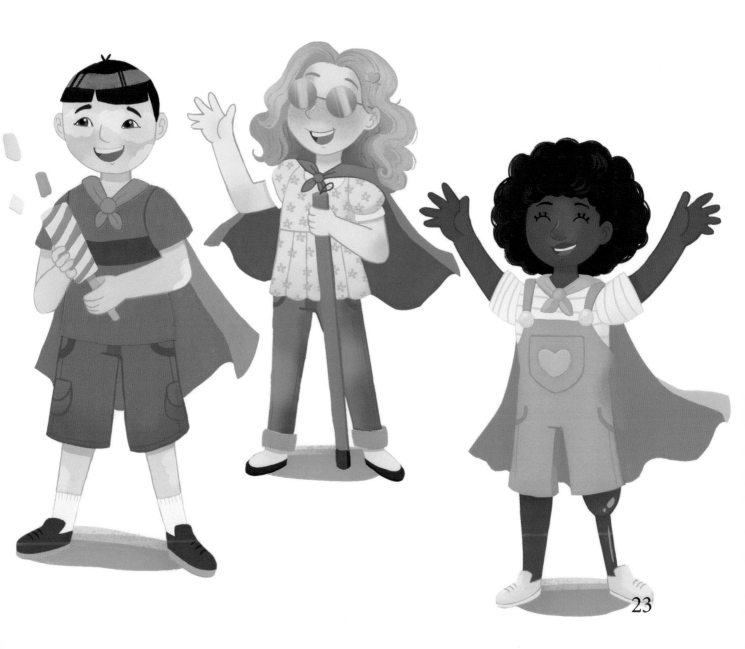

Get to know the *Braver Than I May Know* kids...

Childhood Cancer-Leukemia:
Leukemia is the most common form of cancer in children. The bone marrow makes a large number of abnormal cells that build up and crowd out the healthy blood cells. This prevents the healthy blood cells from doing their normal functions. Pg. 8

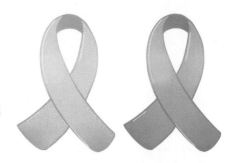

Cystic Fibrosis:
A disorder that causes severe damage to the lungs and digestive system. Cystic Fibrosis can cause severe difficulty breathing and swallowing. Pg. 10

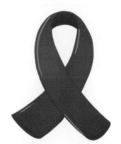

Autism:
A developmental disability that can significantly affect verbal and non-verbal communication and social interaction. Pg. 12

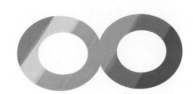

Albinism:
A condition in which the body produces little to no melanin which causes very light skin, hair, and eyes. Albinism can cause vision problems and extreme sensitivity to the sun. Pg. 14

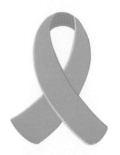

Sickle Cell Disease (also called Sickle Cell Anemia):
A blood disorder that affects red blood cells. This causes the body to make red blood cells that are crescent (or sickle) shape which stick together causing mild to severe pain and discomfort. Pg. 16

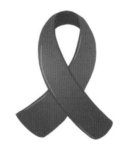

Spina Bifida:
A condition that is present at birth when the spine and spinal cord do not form properly. Spina Bifida can call for the use of crutches, braces, walkers, or wheelchairs depending on the severity. Pg. 18

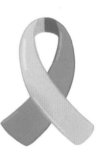

Down Syndrome:
A condition in which a person has an extra chromosome that affects the way the brain and body develop. Pg. 20

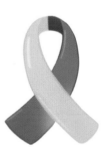

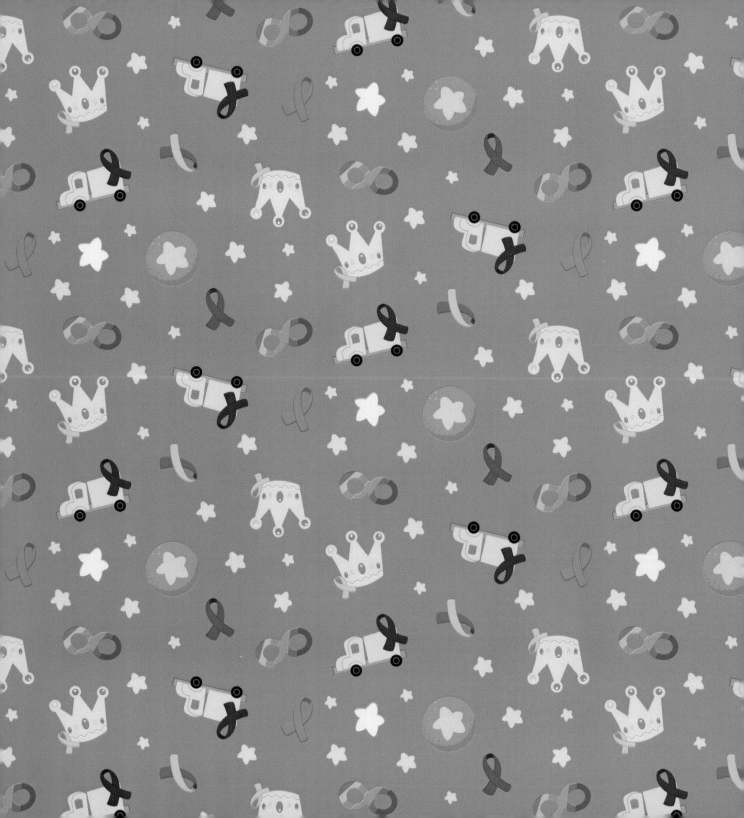